abou

One of Australia's leading be
Walker has worked as bea
including *Woman's Day*, *Dolly* and *She*. She is also a regular contributor
to *GQ*, *Better Health* and the *Sydney Morning Herald*. She has received
several prestigious awards for excellence in journalism.

Shonagh loves to hear from her readers and can be contacted at
the following email address:

contactcellulite@hotmail.com

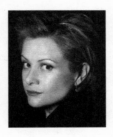

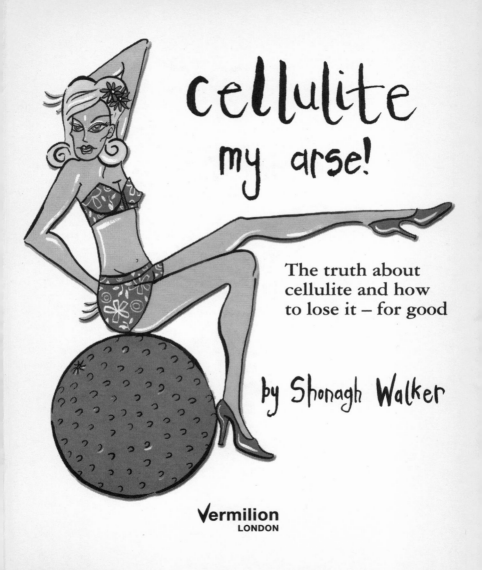

cellulite my arse!

The truth about cellulite and how to lose it – for good

by Shonagh Walker

Vermilion
LONDON

1 3 5 7 9 10 8 6 4 2

Copyright © Shonagh Walker 2001

Shonagh Walker has asserted her right to be identified as the author of this work
in accordance with the Copyright, Designs and Patents Act 1988.

All rights reserved. No part of this publication may be reproduced,
stored in a retrieval system, or transmitted in any form or by any means,
electronic, mechanical, photocopying, recording or otherwise,
without the prior permission of the copyright owner.

First published by HarperCollins Publishers,
A member of HarperCollins (Australia) Pty Limited Group.
This edition published in 2003 by Vermilion,
An imprint of Ebury Press, Random House,
20 Vauxhall Bridge Road, London SW1V 2SA
www.randomhouse.co.uk

Random House Australia (Pty) Limited
20 Alfred Street, Milsons Point, Sydney,
New South Wales 2061, Australia

Random House New Zealand Limited
18 Poland Road, Glenfield,
Auckland 10, New Zealand

Random House South Africa (Pty) Limited
Endulini, 5A Jubilee Road,
Parktown 2193, South Africa

The Random House Group Limited Reg. No. 954009

Text design by Eli Nacson
Text illustrations by Marcus Hay

Papers used by Vermilion are natural, recyclable products
made from wood grown in sustainable forests.

Printed and bound in Great Britain by Mackays of Chatham Plc, Chatham, Kent

A CIP catalogue record for this book is available from the British Library

ISBN 0-09-189043-8

dedication

This book is dedicated to the memory of Julieanne Mee. You probably never had cellulite Juls, but you certainly experienced plenty of life's lumps and bumps. Still, right to the end you met each and every obstacle with tremendous courage, your infectious smile and that wicked sense of humour. You were always an inspiration, and those of us lucky enough to have known you could not help but bask in your rare and beautiful spirit. You were one in a million and you will live on in our hearts and minds forever.

A NOTE FROM THE PUBLISHER

All reasonable care and diligence and attention has been taken in the preparation of material for this book. It is not intended that the information and suggestions made in this book, including but not limited to matters concerning diet, health, exercise and treatment, are to be used by the reader as a substitute for appropriate professional attention and proper medical advice from a qualified health practitioner. The reader should first consult his or her own health practitioner before beginning any exercise, dietary or other program, including any such programs suggested in this book, and the reader should not rely on such information and suggestions in this book without first seeking appropriate medical consultation. The Publisher, author, consultants and editors, or their respective employees and agents, shall not accept responsibility for any injury, loss or damage caused to any person acting or failing to act arising from the material in this book whether or not any such injury, loss or damage is caused by any negligent act, or omission, default or breach of duty by the Publisher, author, consultants and editors, or their respective employees and agents, except as provided by the operation of law.

foreword
by Nene King

I've been on a diet all my life. I've tried The Liver Cleansing Diet, The Israeli Diet, The 9-Eggs-A-Day Diet, The Liquid Protein Diet and The Pritikin Plan. I've lived on cabbage soup for days, and chomped on carrots until my skin turned orange!

I've been to Weight Watchers, Jenny Craig, Gloria Marshall and Overeaters Anonymous. I've filled my freezer with Lean Cuisine and McCain's Healthy Choice low kilojoule meals. Yet my backside still gives new meaning to the word cellulite, and I've had to find a new home for the big boobs I grew after menopause.

My arms are meaty, my ankles thick. I constantly battle with fluid retention and the occasional bloated stomach. Am I not the perfect candidate for Shonagh Walker's new tome *Cellulite My Arse!?*

Thank goodness it doesn't promise a miracle cure! Been there, tried that. There are no miracles in the losing weight department. This little gem of a book provides helpful, sound information, and is designed to relieve women of the problem of cellulite and, more importantly, the low self-esteem issues that tend to accompany it.

I know I should project an image of a smart, sophisticated, woman – someone who has been through hard times and has come out the other end strong and determined and confident. Forget all that fairytale image stuff. If I am overweight, I lose my confidence. If I'm cellulite-bound, I'm depressed. If my jeans are tight, I wallow in self-pity.

In another life I was the group publisher – in other words, the big boss – of the *Australian Women's Weekly*, *Woman's Day*, and *New Weekly* which is now *NW*. I presided over magazines with a yearly profit base of close to $100 million. All those years of giving the women of Australia the best advice and I didn't have the time to heed any of it.

When I began my career as an editor, it was the era of fad diets. I seem to recall I even ran a diet in *Woman's Day* promising weight loss while you slept! These days we are far more sensible. We look for diets with nutritional benefits – all the better if a healthy regimen is coupled with a decent dose of sensible exercise and a guide to boosting self-esteem.

I've known the author Shonagh Walker since those early magical days when *Woman's Day* was the queen of weekly magazines. Shonagh would sit quietly filing transparencies and running herself ragged for grumpy overworked senior editors, but I could see there was more to this bright young thing than a good filing system. She was tenacious and would submit copious beauty features. When a vacancy occurred, I gave Shonagh the opportunity of being beauty editor of *Woman's Day*, Australia's number one weekly magazine. She never looked back. Nor did I – each week she produced entertaining, informative and imaginative beauty pages.

Her knowledge of all things beautiful and healthy, her knowledge of dietary and healthy eating plans was paramount, and I still practise many of her tips today. Don't think this is just another book on cellulite. This is *the* book on cellulite. I guarantee you will lessen the look of those nasty dimples on your bottom and the backs of your legs, and after reading Shonagh's book you'll feel better about yourself. That's what it's all about – self-esteem. By the way, last time I looked, Shonagh was cellulite-less!

contents

acknowledgments

Special thanks to: Nene King and Marie Ussher-Oram for being more than just great bosses – for giving me a start, believing in me and for your constant, unwavering support. To Susie Pitts, Kate Mahon and Pat Ingram for allowing me the opportunity to work on your fabulous titles. To John and Kay for your continual support and generosity. To Cilla for the endless opportunities you throw my way, but more importantly for your friendship and love. To Leon Nacson for lending a helping hand. To Jeannie Bourke at Venustus Beauty and Body Lab, Anna Paredes at Randwick Colon Care Centre and Janie Dallas-Kelly at Air Spa for your knowledge of all things pure and healthy. To Marcus Hay for your wonderful illustrations. To Roberta Marcroft for putting the pieces together and to Alison Urquhart and Karen-Maree Griffiths for gluing them into place.

To Allie Bell, Marty, Max, Lester, Nadya, Deborah, and Magda and Sean for being the best of friends, through good times and bad – dinner is on me, eventually! And to all of my friends who are always there – you all know how much you mean to me.

Finally and especially to my wonderful family, for loving me and believing in me no matter what. Extra special thanks to my beautiful mum for helping me to see myself through a different set of eyes and giving me faith in who I am. I love you up to the sky and the sky after that, etc...

introduction

Let's get the bad news out of the way first. If you're female, chances are that you suffer from cellulite in some way, shape or form. The fact that you're reading this book means you want to get rid of it, or at least get a handle on it. The good news is that you're not alone, and in most cases you can eliminate cellulite, if not certainly reduce the appearance of it.

Throughout my years as a beauty editor on magazines such as *Woman's Day*, *Dolly* and *She*, and now as a freelance beauty and lifestyle writer, one of the most common questions I have been asked is: 'How can I get rid of cellulite?'

It has always amazed me that many of the women who ask this question appear to have the most incredible confidence and sophistication and have been extremely successful in their chosen careers. I have been shocked that, with all their self-assurance, success and beauty, the topic of cellulite would even play on their minds. It just didn't occur to me that it would be such an issue for them with everything else they had going on in their lives. On top of that, I have been stunned that many of these women knew very little about the condition.

But then it struck me that every woman has doubts, concerns and insecurities about her body – even the women we herald as the most beautiful in the world. These women simply know how to project a confident, self-assured public image that deflects the negative aspects of their appearance and draws our attention to the seemingly perfect parts. I say seemingly, because the images that we are presented with through magazines, television and cinema are often achieved with the help of clever fashion tricks, make-up, lighting and camera angles. But more about that later.

The longer I thought about this, the more I became intrigued. Then, one day while I was at the gym, the issue was really driven home. I was packing up my things, getting ready to go home for a night on the sofa, when I overheard two girls talking. One of the girls was a well-known and successful Australian model. Beautiful doesn't even begin to describe her – defined, angular features, enormous eyes, full, pouty lips and a body that most women could only ever dream of possessing. In my eyes, she could not have been more perfect had she been computer generated.

Yet, there she was, looking from behind into the mirror, while she squeezed her thighs and bum between her hands and complained to her friend about the cellulite that was running rampant over the lower half of her body. Since then I've thought a lot about this girl and wondered if her self-doubts have escalated in proportion to her career. I hope not, but I have a feeling they may have. On one hand, it was comforting to know that I wasn't alone with my negative body issues, but on the other, it really showed me that cellulite – and the issues and insecurities that accompany it – is something that concerns every woman.

Which brings me to my reasons for writing this book. I didn't want to write a book that was simply a quick fix, or an overnight solution to cellulite. We all know that doesn't exist. I wanted to offer a sensible approach to a healthier lifestyle and a better self-image that has the added benefit of helping to reduce problem areas and increase your energy levels.

So, over the next seven chapters, I will discuss the causes of cellulite, attempt to dispel some of the common misconceptions surrounding it, then offer safe, non-surgical ways of relieving the problem. I can't promise this will be the perfect solution for everyone, but I can offer some sound and practical advice that, with a little willpower and persistence on your part, should provide relief.

As you read this book, please remember that being beautiful is not about being the thinnest or the shapeliest or even fitting into that little black dress by next Friday night. It's about being the healthiest you can be, maintaining the ideal body weight for your size and frame and being happy with yourself the way you are. More importantly, it is about being fabulous, brilliant and beautiful on the inside.

Best of luck!

Shonagh Walker

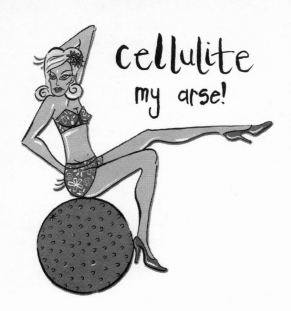

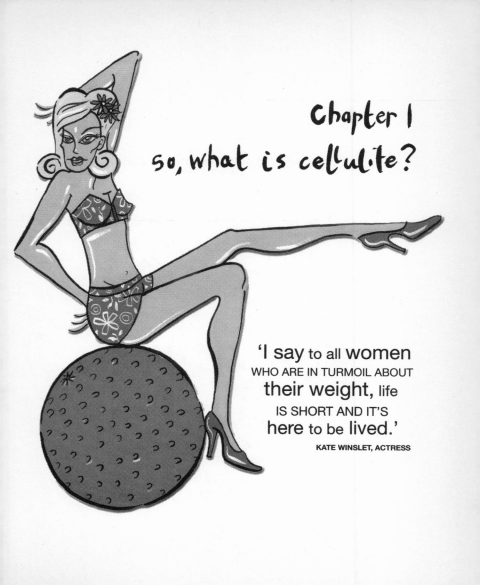

Chapter 1
so, what is cellulite?

'I say to all women
WHO ARE IN TURMOIL ABOUT
their weight, life
IS SHORT AND IT'S
here to be lived.'
KATE WINSLET, ACTRESS

Put simply, cellulite is the name given to the lumpy, irregular fat deposits that are often found on the thighs, hips and buttocks of women. Sometimes, in its most advanced stages, cellulite can also be seen on the stomach, breasts and arms. It doesn't matter who you are, if you're female and past puberty then you may be prone to cellulite and will probably experience it at some stage in your life. It may comfort you to know that this includes the supermodels and actresses we are confronted with every time we turn on the television or open a magazine. That's right – rich or poor, short or tall, fat or thin, curvy or lanky, young or old – anyone can have cellulite.

Thankfully, cellulite is something we can all control, and it doesn't have to be something that keeps you away from the beach, or lowers your self-esteem.

how bad is the problem?

dimples you don't want

Cellulite, as you will know if you have it, has a dimpled appearance on the skin that often resembles orange peel or the surface of a golf ball. This dimpling is not always specifically related to cellulite. It's actually directly related to the honeycomb-like distribution of fat in women. In cases of cellulite, the orange peel effect is associated with poorly functioning blood vessels within this 'honeycomb' – if blood vessels are weak and sluggish, toxins can quickly accumulate making it difficult for the body to burn fat in cellulite-affected areas. However, before we delve into its causes, it's important to note that there are four different stages of cellulite. In order to find a solution to your problem, you must first determine what stage your cellulite is at.

what stage of cellulite do i have?

1. ARE YOU AGED?

A. Under 30.

B. Between 30 and 35.

C. Between 35 and 40.

D. 40 years or more.

2. ARE YOU OR HAVE YOU BEEN?

A. On the contraceptive pill.

B. Pregnant with your first child.

C. Pregnant with your second (or other) child.

D. Menopausal and on Hormone Replacement Therapy.

3. WHEN YOU LOOK AT YOUR THIGHS, HIPS AND BOTTOM, DOES THE SKIN APPEAR?

A. Smooth and even in tone, with slight dimpling when you squeeze it.

B. Smooth and even, with some dimpled areas that are blotchy in tone.

C. Quite dimpled and blotchy in many areas, with a blue tinge over the complexion.

D. Very dimpled and blotchy, with a blue-grey tinge covering most of the surface.

4. WHEN YOU TOUCH YOUR THIGHS, HIPS AND BOTTOM, WHAT DOES IT FEEL LIKE?

A. Fairly smooth, with an even temperature.

B. Smooth and even in temperature, aside from a few areas affected by dimples, which are occasionally cold, clammy and slightly spongy.

C. Cold, clammy and spongy in many areas.

D. Spongy all over, with a very cold temperature and clammy consistency.

5. WOULD YOU SAY YOU EXERCISE?

A. Frequently, at least three to four times per week.

B. Moderately, about once or twice per week.

C. Rarely, perhaps once or twice a month.

D. Never, maybe once or twice each year.

6. HOW FREQUENTLY DO YOU EAT FRESH FRUIT AND VEGETABLES?

A. Daily, at least two or three serves.

B. Every second or third day.

C. Rarely, you seldom have the time to prepare a meal.

D. Never, you eat on the run and it's usually whatever is in the takeaway food store at the time.

7. HOW OFTEN DO YOU EAT JUNK FOOD?

A. Rarely, perhaps once every two or three months.

B. At least once or twice a month.

C. Perhaps two or three times a week.

D. Almost on a daily basis.

check what's on
your table

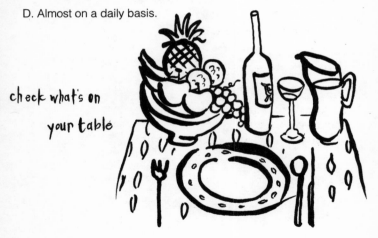

cellulite my arse!

8. DO YOU SMOKE?

A. Never.

B. Socially, maybe on Friday nights or over the weekend.

C. In the evenings, most nights of the week.

D. Every day, sometimes a packet or more each day.

9. YOU DRINK ALCOHOL:

A. Only on special occasions.

B. On weekends only.

C. Three or four nights a week.

D. Every night, and more on the weekends.

10. YOUR INTAKE OF WATER IS:

A. At least one or two litres each day.

B. Half a litre to one litre every day.

C. One litre every second day.

D. Perhaps one litre each week.

11. YOU DRINK COFFEE, TEA OR SOFT DRINK:

A. Very rarely, perhaps once or twice a month.

B. Only a few times each week.

C. Once a day.

D. Regularly throughout the day.

results

Before you read your results, please note that this is merely a guide to determine the stage of cellulite you have. It is possible that your answers may be an equal number of As and Bs, or that more than one answer in a question applies to you. If this is the case, it is possible that you are 'in-between' stages, ie: Stage One progressing into Stage Two.

It may also be that you answered mostly As, but you still seem to have very severe cellulite. If this is the case, you may need to see your GP, who can recommend a nutritionist and fitness/exercise expert who can tailor a program to your individual and specific needs. Or you may have answered mostly Ds, and yet have virtually no cellulite at all, in which case you will be the envy of all your friends. Cellulite, while something we are all prone to, is a very individual thing, so please just use this as a reference point, along with a good dose of common sense, in determining the seriousness of your condition.

MOSTLY A – STAGE ONE

If you found yourself circling mostly As, then it's likely that you have only mild cellulite or Stage One. Women who experience Stage One cellulite are likely to be under thirty, with a fairly active lifestyle and a relatively healthy diet. The appearance of cellulite in this stage is quite compact, and while you could notice some dimpled areas, it's likely that you will only notice the problem when you squeeze the flesh in your hands. Contributors to the condition in this early stage could be the contraceptive pill, which can increase oestrogen levels, or perhaps a genetic predisposition to the condition. We will explore both of these in more detail in Chapter Two.

MOSTLY B – STAGE TWO

Mostly Bs indicates Stage Two cellulite, which is mild to problematic. The appearance of cellulite is noticeable, however it is compact and localised rather than covering an expansive area. There will be a blotchiness to the skin tone in these areas, and they can feel spongy and clammy to the touch. Generally, this stage is experienced by women between the ages of thirty and thirty-five, who for the most part have a fairly healthy diet, but often reach for convenience or fast foods, and may slack off on exercise. Again, taking the contraceptive pill or pregnancy can contribute to the problem due to an increase in oestrogen levels. We will discuss the relationship between oestrogen and cellulite in greater detail in Chapter Two.

MOSTLY C – STAGE THREE

If you found yourself circling all Cs, then you are likely to have Stage Three cellulite, which can be more of a problem. The cellulite-affected areas will be of greater expanse and will be quite noticeable over the thighs, hips and buttocks. Skin will have less elasticity, can often appear blotchy and spongelike, and will have a grey or blue discolouration due to poor circulation. The skin can be cold and clammy to touch and won't spring back quickly when pressed. Stage Three usually affects women aged between thirty-five and forty who have been on the Pill, have had children, or may have experienced pregnancy. These women are more likely to eat on the run and often reach for the wrong types of foods. There are many more factors contributing to this stage, all of which we will uncover in the next chapter.

MOSTLY D – STAGE FOUR

If you circled mostly Ds, then you probably have Stage Four cellulite. This stage is the most advanced, and while it certainly isn't life-threatening, it can be extremely uncomfortable and painful for those who experience it. It is very noticeable, and can often be seen through clothing. It is likely to occur in women aged over forty who have had children, have experienced menopause or are on Hormone Replacement Therapy, although this is not always the case. A poor diet and less than ideal exercise habits do contribute, but there are many other factors involved that we will delve into in Chapter Two.

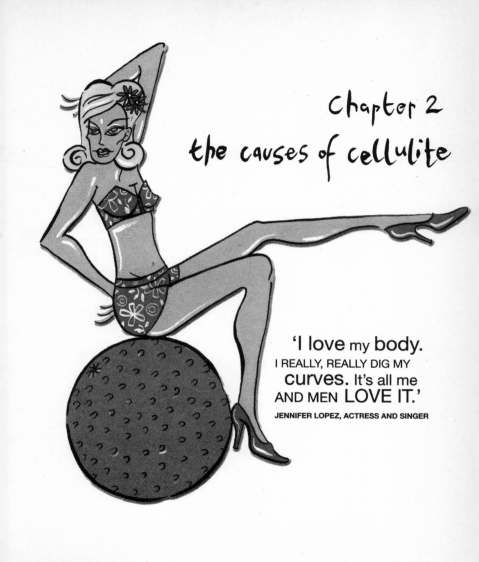

Chapter 2
the causes of cellulite

'I love my body. I REALLY, REALLY DIG MY curves. It's all me AND MEN LOVE IT.'
JENNIFER LOPEZ, ACTRESS AND SINGER

*t*here are many different theories about the causes of cellulite, however all seem to lead to the following conclusion: cellulite is the direct result of poorly functioning lymphatic and circulatory systems, brought on by a variety of contributing factors.

cellulite — the real deal

Cellulite is not your everyday, ordinary fat that can be controlled with sensible eating habits and exercise alone. It also can't be treated simply by rubbing in a cream each day, or having a regular lymphatic drainage massage — it must be treated holistically and that means changing your thought processes, re-analysing your lifestyle and making sensible, healthy choices. In order to do this, you need to know all the facts.

Unlike regular stores of fat, cellulite cannot be accessed and used by the body as an energy source. This is because it is essentially fat that has become trapped within the connective tissues in the affected areas. Let me explain.

The reason women and not men are affected by cellulite is that the compartments that hold our fat cells differ in shape. In men, these compartments are square in shape, so they all sit in a nice, uniformed way, regardless of how thin or overweight a man is.

In women, these compartments are elongated and protrude closer to the surface, especially on the hips, thighs and buttocks. They are held together by connective fibres that resemble the shape of a honeycomb. If fat and fluids accumulate in these compartments, they tend to bulge out and press against the connective tissue, creating the external lumpiness.

Over time, this bulging can become severe enough to restrict the blood supply to these areas, trapping the fat. Because the fat is now trapped, it is not available to be accessed as an energy source, which is why no amount of exercise alone can reduce the appearance of cellulite.

As we age, or as the stages of cellulite progress, these elongated compartments of fat cells expand and the cellulite becomes more visible. Meanwhile, the 'honeycomb' or supportive fibres tighten, adding to the bulges. In very severe stages of cellulite, circulation is dramatically slowed down, accounting for the cold, clammy and spongy feeling. Nerve endings may also become compressed and tender, which is why women with advanced stages of cellulite can often suffer pain from the condition.

the lymphatic and circulatory systems

The lymphatic and circulatory systems work side by side, ensuring that your body runs efficiently. They control the oxygenation and nutrition of every cell in your body, the digestion of food and the absorption of nutrients, as well as the elimination of wastes and toxins. In particular, the lymphatic system works closely with blood circulation to flush impurities through the intestinal tract and out of the body. Should these systems become sluggish, for whatever reason, then toxins and wastes will not be eliminated efficiently. Consequently, the blood and lymphatic vessels can weaken and allow fluids and toxins to leak into the surrounding tissues. For reasons that will be explained when we discuss oestrogen, this seems to occur mainly in the hip, thigh and buttock regions.

In short, anything that hinders circulation and lymph drainage will contribute or add to the condition of cellulite. This can range from high levels of oestrogen, to poor eating habits, lack of exercise, smoking and even drinking coffee.

the cellulite/oestrogen connection

The female hormone oestrogen is now thought to be a major contributor to the problem of cellulite. Among its many functions, oestrogen stores and distributes fat within the female body. Think of it as Mother Nature's way of preparing us for hardship. In times gone by, when famine threatened, women could carry on breastfeeding their babies thanks to the extra fuel supplies in their bodies that were localised in the hip, thigh and buttock areas. These days in the Western world, we are fortunate enough for famine not to be a threat, but oestrogen does not recognise this, and so it carries on with the function of fat and energy storage.

It's also thought that oestrogen increases the permeability of the blood and lymphatic vessels in cellulite-prone areas, allowing fluids to leak into the surrounding tissues. This creates the congestion that restricts blood flow and circulation, and eventually traps the fats and fluids. The spongy feel and appearance of cellulite is probably due to this fluid excess, while the restricted blood flow and circulation accounts for the cold, clammy feeling of the skin. This poor circulation also means that the cells in this area become undernourished, which in turn leaves the skin looking dry, dull and bluish-grey in tone.

High oestrogen levels can intensify, as well as contribute to, the problem of cellulite. This is why cellulite often appears with the onset of puberty and may become worse when a woman starts taking the contraceptive pill or becomes pregnant. While menopause may slightly relieve the condition, Hormone Replacement Therapies may also add to the condition.

diet and nutrition

Every single cell in your body requires energy to stay healthy and strong and to function optimally, and this includes the cells that make up your digestive, circulatory and lymphatic systems. When you are not feeding your body with the correct nutrients to sustain these systems, they become sluggish, and impurities, toxins and wastes are not eliminated efficiently.

A diet high in refined, processed, junk or fatty foods will contribute to poor circulatory functioning purely because it does nothing to encourage the body's natural digestive or metabolic processes. These foods contain very few vitamins or minerals and are so refined that they are able to pass through the lining of the stomach with very little effort on the part of your digestive system. As a result, these systems become lazy, and the more you indulge in this type of diet, the slower and more sluggish these systems become. In time, this leads to the build up of toxins and wastes that can trigger the onset of cellulite.

caffeine and sugary soft drinks

Too many caffeinated, sugary drinks can have the same effect on your metabolism as a poor diet, but for a different reason. Drinks that are high in caffeine or sugar have the ability to boost energy levels and, for a time, your metabolism. This is why you often feel buzzed or even a little jittery after a strong cup of coffee.

However, in the tradition of what goes up must come down, you inevitably crash from this high, bringing your mood, your energy levels and your metabolism to an even lower level than they were to begin with.

excess caffeine can make things worse

lack of exercise

Regular exercise contributes to a fit, healthy body – one where all bodily functions are working at their peak, muscles are toned and the cardiovascular system is strong and vital. If exercise is teamed with a sensible diet, circulation and metabolism will function efficiently, as will the digestive and waste elimination processes. Conversely, lack of exercise contributes to sluggish circulation and waste elimination, and toxin build-up, all of which contribute to cellulite.

lack of hydration

Our bodies are made up of around seventy per cent water, so it makes sense that we rely on a regular intake of water in order to sustain normal bodily functions. We lose around two to three litres of water each day through sweat and urine, and these require constant replacement. Insufficient water intake can once again result in poor circulation and a sluggish metabolism, and will contribute to cellulite.

drink plenty of pure water

smoking

Aside from the innumerable dangers associated with the habit, smoking can directly lead to the onset of cellulite. The smoke you inhale with each cigarette is loaded with poisons and toxins, which add to the accumulation of toxins in your body. Furthermore, smoking dramatically restricts the circulation of blood, inhibiting the correct nutrition and oxygenation of the cells, and slowing down the lymphatic and waste elimination systems.

Consequently, toxins, wastes and fluids accumulate and cellulite may result.

alcohol

Excessive alcohol intake and alcohol abuse can lead to a poorly functioning liver. The chief functions of the liver are to help the body digest and use food, and to help purify the blood of wastes and poisons. Clearly, if the liver is not functioning efficiently it cannot effectively remove these wastes, which leads to a build up of toxins. Alcohol also has an extremely dehydrating effect on the body, which in turn causes the circulatory system to slow down in an effort to keep the body hydrated.

constipation

Usually a result of a poor diet, constipation is often thought to contribute to cellulite because it allows the toxins and wastes to remain in the body rather than flushing them out via the alimentary canal. In every twenty-four hour period, an adult body eliminates billions of dead cells and must also eliminate the chemicals and toxins we take in from food, air, water and the environment. If these toxins cannot pass through the colon because it is inactive or sluggish, they stay in the body and can ultimately affect the efficiency of major purifying organs such as the liver and kidneys.

stress

Stress is a major contributing factor in many modern day illnesses and conditions, and cellulite is no exception. When under stress, our bodies experience what is known as a flight or fight reaction, where the blood is directed to the arms and legs in preparation for flight – running away from the situation, or fight – staying to face the situation, and if necessary going into battle.

It dates back to prehistoric man, when the greatest threats he had to encounter were predators in the wild. Other responses in such situations are a tightening of the muscles, shallowness of breath and a rush of adrenaline. All of these factors take energy away from the circulatory and digestive systems, causing sluggish circulation and, in turn, the build up of toxins and fats in the body.

Many of us also deal with stress by eating, and usually the first thing we grab is 'comfort food', something that may taste great but that is not necessarily great for you. These will also give you a quick energy fix, which may make you feel slightly better for a while. The problem is that these foods are usually high in fat and sugar, as well as impurities and toxins that may be harmful to the body.

genetics

While there is no conclusive proof that you will develop cellulite if your mother did, it is generally accepted that a genetic predisposition is a contributing factor. Should you have a family member with the problem, it may be wise to take precautionary steps, as outlined in Chapter Four, to lessen your chances of developing it.

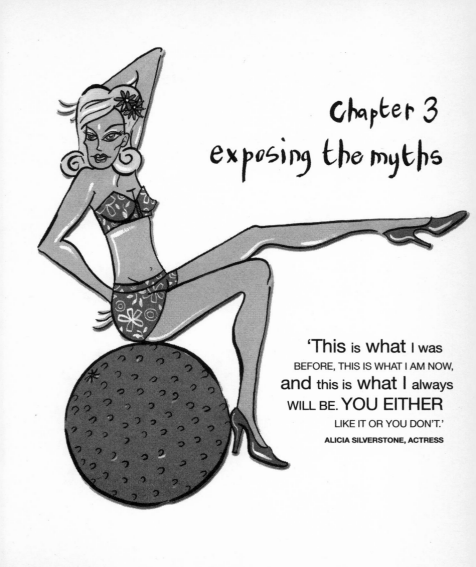

Chapter 3
exposing the myths

'This is what I was BEFORE, THIS IS WHAT I AM NOW, and this is what I always WILL BE. YOU EITHER LIKE IT OR YOU DON'T.'
ALICIA SILVERSTONE, ACTRESS

there are many myths and untruths surrounding cellulite, and before we go any further it's best to dispel any confusion and set the record straight.

myth:
Cellulite only happens to fat or overweight people.

truth:
Even very slim women can have areas of cellulite on their thighs, buttocks and hips. Surprisingly, they can even be in quite advanced stages.

myth:
Strict dieting will eliminate cellulite.

truth:
Dieting alone cannot get rid of cellulite, in fact crash dieting may even make the condition worse as it dramatically slows the metabolism. What occurs when you deprive the body of food is that your system

goes into famine mode, storing fat as an energy resource, which is why you can actually gain weight by crash dieting. Along with this reservoir reaction, your circulatory system slows down, which means you are not efficiently eliminating the wastes and toxins your body needs to flush out, resulting in a more serious problem than the one you began with!

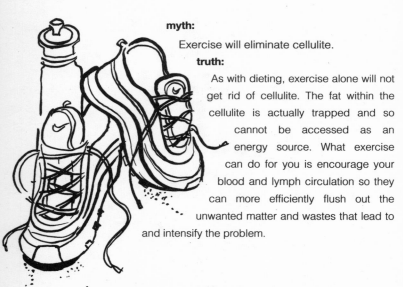

myth:

Exercise will eliminate cellulite.

truth:

As with dieting, exercise alone will not get rid of cellulite. The fat within the cellulite is actually trapped and so cannot be accessed as an energy source. What exercise can do for you is encourage your blood and lymph circulation so they can more efficiently flush out the unwanted matter and wastes that lead to and intensify the problem.

regular exercise will stimulate circulation

myth:

Cellulite is not serious and can't get any worse.

truth:

While it is certainly not life-threatening, if you don't take action against the appearance of cellulite, it can get worse. If it gets beyond Stage Three, it can be extremely difficult to do anything about, and may even become a source of discomfort or pain.

myth:

Cellulite is a natural part of ageing.

truth:

Cellulite does intensify with age, however it often has a lot to do with the loss of skin elasticity and firmness, which can make the appearance more apparent. The good news is that you can do something about its undesirable appearance – you don't have to accept it.

myth:

Cellulite is a completely curable condition and can be eliminated over time.

truth:

It is really only possible to eliminate the early stages of cellulite. Stage One and Stage Two can be diminished with the proper practices (see Chapters Four and Five). Stage Three is slightly more difficult to relieve, but it can certainly be improved. If you have cellulite that is in Stage Four, it is unlikely you will ever completely be rid of the condition, however, there are still certain steps that you can take to improve the general appearance of your skin.

myth:

Massage can eliminate cellulite.

truth:

Vigorous massage such as deep tissue techniques can actually intensify the condition, especially if they are not performed correctly. The harsh pummelling and crunching involved can weaken the underlying support structures, increase the flow of wastes to the area and make the swelling of the tissues worse.

If you want to use massage as a relief, opt for lymphatic drainage techniques that use specialised, gentle movements designed specifically to encourage a sluggish lymph system into a healthy state.

gentle stimulating massage can help

myth:

Cellulite is simply a fancy name for fat.

truth:

Fat is fat and is something that can be accessed by the metabolism as an energy source, which is why a low fat diet and exercise are particularly useful for losing weight. Cellulite is not only made up of fat, but also toxins, lymph fluid, and wastes that are all trapped within the support structure beneath the skin (see Chapter Two). As such, cellulite cannot readily be used as an energy source by the body and a good deal of effort is required to lessen its appearance.

myth:

There is no cream, body wrap or salon treatment that can help lessen the appearance of cellulite.

truth:

While these treatments certainly won't eliminate the problem on their own, they may assist in nurturing the surface of the skin, leaving it feeling softer and more supple. They can also impart a feeling of wellbeing that may help to improve self-worth and confidence, making the problem seem less significant to the sufferer.

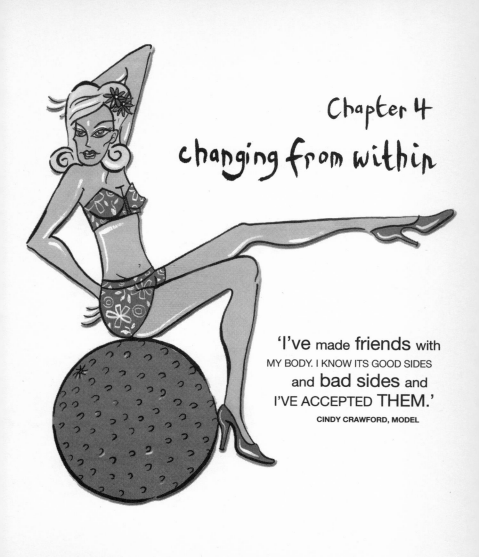

Chapter 4
changing from within

'I've made friends with MY BODY. I KNOW ITS GOOD SIDES and bad sides and I'VE ACCEPTED THEM.'

CINDY CRAWFORD, MODEL

beauty is only skin deep. Beauty comes from within. You are what you eat. They're clichés you've heard a thousand times over, yet never have they made more sense than when applied to cellulite. You can rub on expensive creams, be massaged or wrapped in seaweed every day of the week, but unless you take steps to encourage your circulation from the inside, you won't ever completely rid yourself of cellulite. In this chapter, we'll explore some of the inside solutions.

first things first

To reduce the appearance of cellulite, aim to do things that will strengthen the tissues in the cellulite-affected areas, encourage your circulation and metabolism, and flush out toxins in order to cleanse the systems within your body. It's also important to nourish and condition cellulite-affected areas in order to strengthen the supportive structures and loosen the restricted circulation.

Essentially, you need to work towards increasing the blood flow in the veins and arteries, and the activity of the lymphatic vessels. It sounds terribly difficult, but it's really not! It's all about making the right choices as far as what you eat and drink, and taking in regular exercise. In Chapter Six, we outline a detoxifying two-week cleansing diet devised with the help of naturopath Anna Paredes from the Randwick Colon Care Centre in Sydney. This is a very useful starting point on your journey to a new you, because it gently coaxes the body into 'flush-out' mode.

As you are working to increase circulation and improve lymphatic function, work on increasing your metabolic rate (that's the rate at which your body burns food and stored energy), so that once the restricted areas can be accessed, the fat that has been trapped can be metabolised. Gentle yet challenging regular exercise is the most sensible way to do this.

By improving blood and lymph circulation it makes sense that blocked areas can once again receive nourishment, making it possible for the trapped fat to be used as an energy source. And by increasing the rate at which your body burns energy – your metabolic rate – you will increase your chances of reducing the appearance of your cellulite. Here are some effective methods of achieving these goals.

weighty issues

Not everyone who has cellulite is overweight, and being overweight is certainly not the cause of cellulite, however excess weight is often associated with the incidence of cellulite.

Remember that it is crucial not to try crash or fad diets. Most doctors and nutritionists flatly state that these types of weight loss methods only compound a weight problem and tamper with your metabolism. Crash diets simply lower the metabolism as your body believes that it is in a time of famine and the metabolism slows down in order to conserve energy reserves.

A sensible eating plan, combined with regular exercise that works the cardiovascular system and tones the body, is the only way to reduce weight and maintain a healthy body weight.

choose your food wisely

The type of food you consume is undoubtedly more important than how much food you eat. While too much of any food can lead to weight problems, it's important to eat a well-balanced diet that includes at least three medium-sized meals each day. I guess the key is to think about everything you put in your mouth, and to look at food as fuel for your

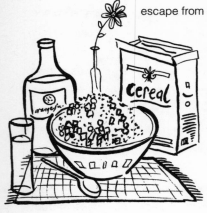

body, rather than a reward, a pick-me-up or an escape from boredom.

In cases of cellulite, where your blood and lymph systems have become sluggish, it's wise to opt for foods that can assist in stimulating bodily functions, such as high fibre foods like fruit, vegetables and whole-grain cereals. Try as well to include foods that will stimulate the detoxifying process, such as beetroot, celery, cucumber and onions.

eating a healthy good-sized breakfast will boost your metabolism

Where possible, try to eat raw rather than cooked fruits and vegetables. A fruit-only breakfast is a great way to start each day. It's light, filling and encourages the body's systems to wake up without overloading them. Mix a few different kinds of fruit in a bowl for your breakfast. A freshly peeled paw paw, a slice of pineapple, a handful of strawberries, a kiwi fruit, an apple – they all taste great, will fill you up and have plenty of essential vitamins and minerals that will nourish your system and assist in cleansing away toxins.

If you find it really difficult to eat your vegetables raw, steam them very lightly so that they are still a little crunchy when served. That way you will preserve their nutritional value. Season them with lemon juice and herbs, rather than lashings of butter and salt. Instead of making a large piece of steak the focus of your meal, halve the size of your meat and increase the amount of your vegetables. Make the vegetables the focus and include as many different colours as possible on your plate – a lovely fresh red beetroot, a yellow squash, a few green snow peas and an orange capsicum. If you look at your vegetables in terms of colours and try to eat at least four or five different coloured vegetables each day, you are well on your way to improving your diet.

Always choose fresh, natural fruits and vegetables – avoid the tinned variety that may have hidden preservatives, sugars and salts – and try to opt for organic selections that are free from herbicides and pesticides. Aim to leave the skin on your fruit and vegetables as much of the nutritional and fibre content can be found there. For the same reason, try to eat the core and the pips.

You may opt to follow a vegetarian or vegan diet. If so, it is very important that you include foods that will give you essential nutrients such as calcium and iron. This means swapping to soy substitutes and eating plenty of legumes, green leafy vegetables, nuts and whole-grain cereals. If at any point you feel that your diet is lacking, your energy levels are depleted or your skin takes on a grey pallor, see your GP and a nutritionist immediately for dietary advice.

If you do eat meat, chicken and eggs, opt for organic, farm-raised choices, which are free from hormones, preservatives and chemicals. Fish is an excellent source of protein and essential fatty acids that are great for the skin. Always grill any meat choice, rather than fry, to maintain nutritional value and to allow as much fat to drip away as possible.

Try not to eat meat, chicken or fish too late in the day – lunchtime is ideal. It's often recommended that women with cellulite avoid eating large amounts of protein, especially in the late afternoon or evening, as unused protein can put a strain on the lymph system.

Avoid refined carbohydrates such as white rice, white bread and white pasta. They can cause gas and may coagulate in the digestive tract and be difficult and slow to metabolise. Always opt for wholemeal or whole-grain alternatives that are high in fibre and will stimulate the digestive system. I like to think of fibre as a workout for your internal organs and digestive system. The more roughage you ingest, the harder your internal organs have to work to digest the food and gain benefits from it, which makes these organs fit and healthy and boosts the metabolism and circulatory system. You could liken the effect to working out at the gym to tone and strengthen your muscles.

Finally and very importantly, before you embark on any new or radically different eating plan, always consult your GP and a qualified, reputable nutritionist or naturopath. Every individual has certain needs that differ from another. These professionals can monitor any particular medical requirements that you may have, and advise as to whether a certain eating plan is safe for you and suited to your needs.

reduce salt intake

A high salt intake can intensify the problems of fluid retention and bloating, as well as put a strain on the blood and circulatory systems. In many cases, it can cause high blood pressure and put a strain on the walls of the veins and major arteries.

Enjoying the natural tastes of foods is clearly the best way to go, however it can take a while to wean yourself off salt. Try flavouring food with herbs, black pepper, chilli or lemon juice, or use natural alternatives such as the Dr A. Vogel blends of herbs and seasonings. It's interesting to note that people who smoke have a lesser sense of taste than non-smokers, which often accounts for a high salt intake. People who have given up smoking have often reported that the taste of food is intensified, in which case they add less seasoning to their meals.

boosting your metabolism

Your metabolism has a direct effect on the amount of fat you store and often the circulatory system within the body. Some people can eat as much as they like and whatever they want and remain slim, while others pile on weight simply by smelling food. If you have a sluggish metabolism, wise ways of boosting it include gentle cardiovascular exercise, preferably first thing in the morning, eating a larger breakfast followed by a smaller lunch and even smaller dinner, grazing on fruit or raw vegetables throughout the day, increasing your intake of fibre and drinking large amounts of filtered water.

stop smoking

Aside from myriad health risks, smoking can contribute to and compound the problem of cellulite as it restricts circulation and prevents the body from being properly nourished. If you have trouble giving up ask your doctor for help, or contact your local Quit Line.

watch what you drink

Watching what you drink doesn't just involve alcohol, although it is wise to cut back as much as possible as consuming excessive amounts can impair liver function and drastically dehydrate the body.

If you must indulge, limit yourself to one glass of red wine per day, as it contains powerful anti-oxidants that are actually very good for you.

Drinks such as coffee, tea, caffeine-containing soft drinks, and even diet soft drinks that may contain caffeine, can all have a detrimental effect on the body. They add unwanted toxins to the system, can slow down the metabolism and circulatory system and leave you feeling tired, listless and fatigued.

Smart and tasty alternatives include green tea, dandelion tea, and herbal teas (organic varieties are best). Hot water with lemon and ginger is also extremely calming and cleansing as it assists with the removal of toxins and

swap caffeinated drinks for cleansing herbal tea

peppermint

wastes from the body by encouraging the liver and kidneys to flush out impurities. It is also imperative that you drink plenty of fresh, pure water on a daily basis. You lose two to three litres of water from your body every day through sweat and dehydration, so this needs to be replaced in order to sustain proper bodily functions, in particular blood and lymph circulation.

colonic irrigation

Princess Diana was said to have been an avid fan of this practice, and while it certainly isn't everyone's cup of tea, many find the benefits to be invaluable. It can reduce bloating and gas, and is thought to be able to lower the risk of intestinal disease.

Toxins can build up in the colon wall in much the same way as plaque builds up on your teeth. Basically, what colonic irrigation does is hydrate the colon and allow built-up faecal matter, mucus and toxins to dislodge and be flushed out of the system. While it may not suit the very shy, most reputable practitioners will immediately make you feel at ease, relaxed and safe. Always try to visit a centre that is clean and uses disposable hoses and tubes. The actual process can be as comfortable or uncomfortable as you make it – it all depends on your diet and lifestyle. If you haven't slept well, have eaten a lot of sugar, refined carbohydrates, fats and salt, or had a lot of alcohol, soft drink, coffee or tea to drink during the week before your treatment, you may find that your irrigation is particularly uncomfortable due to gas build-up. On the other hand, plenty of sleep and a sensible diet of brown rice, fresh fruits and vegetables and fish will allow the treatment to clear away toxins with very little discomfort.

Generally, it is recommended that for your first treatment, you have one session each week for three weeks, then one every six months after that. Those who have experienced colonic irrigation generally rave about the effect it has on clearing the whites of their eyes, adding luminosity to their skin and assisting them in adopting a healthier lifestyle.

ashtanga yoga

A dynamic, challenging form of Hatha Yoga, this ancient type of yoga works the body and mind on many different levels. It is renowned for its mental, emotional and spiritual benefits, however it is also brilliant for improving the strength, flexibility and fitness of the physical body. It improves balance, grace and posture, and firms and tones almost every muscle in the body.

You only need to look at the physiques of its celebrity devotees to know that it works. Madonna attributes her post-baby body to regular sessions of Ashtanga Yoga, and Demi Moore has long been practising it, as have Gwyneth Paltrow, Sting and Woody Harrelson. Ashtanga is especially useful for conditions such as cellulite, as it not only shapes and tones muscles, but works directly on improving the cardiovascular and blood circulatory systems. This is due to the synchronisation of deep, forceful breaths with many forward bending, strength enhancing postures that aid in digestion and toxin removal.

You should be able to find a reputable teacher by phoning around yoga centres in your area, however make sure you check their credentials thoroughly. It is a good idea to ask how long they have been teaching and find out where they studied before you sign up. Ashtanga Yoga is a very specific and specialised discipline, and should only be taught by well-trained and well-informed teachers. Usually, a properly trained Ashtanga teacher will have been to the Ashtanga Yoga Institute in Mysore, India, and trained under Sri K. Pattabhi Jois who helped to develop the discipline of Ashtanga as we know it today.

Ashtanga Yoga improves fitness, tone and circulation and helps detoxify

breathing and relaxation techniques

The importance of time out and relaxation cannot be underestimated. Simple meditations and relaxation techniques can be practised anywhere and will help to reduce anxiety and clear the thought processes. Something as simple as burning your favourite incense or an aromatherapy oil such as lavender, rose or ylang ylang can reduce stress levels enormously.

The following is a simple, effective technique that I practise frequently if I'm stressed, annoyed, or having trouble getting to sleep. Start by closing your eyes and inhaling deeply. Hold your breath for a few seconds and, as you do, imagine that all the tension, anxiety, sadness or negative thoughts and emotions within you are grouping together in the held breath that is sitting in the bottom of your lungs. Imagine them as a black, toxic smoke, swirling inside you, waiting to be let out. Now allow your breath to flow out of your nostrils. Ensure the breath out is long and extended. As it leaves your nostrils, imagine the toxic black smoke in your lungs leaving through your nostrils and taking these mind toxins with it. As you take your next deep breath in, imagine that the air entering your nostrils is a pure, beautiful, shimmering golden light that is flowing through your body and entering every cell. Repeat this three or four times until your anxiety and stress have passed.

Finally, learn how to breathe deeply and smoothly. Far too often we take in rapid, shallow breaths, leaving our bodies depleted of oxygen and running on empty. Make a conscious effort to breathe deeply by setting aside certain times of the day to practise breathing techniques such as this one. After a while you will find that you slip into a habit of deep breathing automatically.

detoxify your mind

Remember that it is one thing to detoxify and exercise your body, but you also have to do the same thing to your mind. Try to change your way of thinking from the negative to the positive whenever possible. Remember that if you think that you can achieve something, you will. If you start thinking that you can't achieve anything, it's highly unlikely that you're ever going to.

Detoxifying your mind isn't only about believing in yourself, although that's one huge step! It's about training your mind to choose to reach for an apple instead of a chocolate bar, to steam your potatoes instead of deep frying them, and to walk to work instead of taking the bus. Do indulge every now and then, but try to do it in moderation. Instead of having the large popcorn at the movies, have the small and buy a bottle of water instead of a fizzy, sugary soft drink.

Detoxifying your mind is also about learning to manage stress and emotional situations in a clear and rational way. Mind toxins appear in the form of anxiety, emotional upheaval, daily thought processes and external stimuli that has a subliminal effect on your stress levels. All of these things contribute to many of the illnesses we see in today's society, such as Chronic Fatigue Syndrome and conditions such as cellulite. Take time out for yourself, learn how to relax and enjoy life, and spend time with your loved ones as much as you can. Remember that work will always be there tomorrow – your opportunities to be with friends and family, have an adventure, and live your life to the fullest may not – so make the most of them while you can.

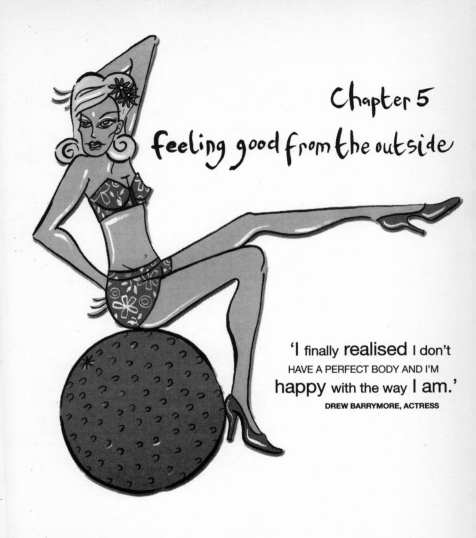

Chapter 5
feeling good from the outside

'I finally **realised** I don't HAVE A PERFECT BODY AND I'M **happy** with the way **I am.**'
DREW BARRYMORE, ACTRESS

*t*reating cellulite from the inside, in conjunction with exercise, is without a doubt the best way to tackle it, but it can often take from two to four months before you notice a radical difference. In the meantime, don't become disheartened – spoil yourself! A few regular skin-maintenance regimes can help to improve the skin's smoothness, enhance its tone, and may even assist in making the problem slightly less noticeable, which will ultimately make you feel better about yourself.

dry body brushing

Your skin is your body's largest excretory organ, and many toxins are released through it via sweat. If dead cells are allowed to accumulate on the surface of the skin, it becomes difficult for these toxins to be released, leading to dull, dry skin and often blemishes. A minimum of twice a week dry body brushing helps to maintain healthy skin by sloughing away the build-up of dead cells.

As body brushing works in synchronisation with the circulatory system, it is also very useful in stimulating the removal of toxins via the lymphatic glands. Whether it alone is useful in the removal of cellulite is doubtful, however the positive effect it has on the skin in general is one that can't be ignored.

Prior to your morning shower, use a natural, firm-bristled body brush on dry skin and, starting at your left foot, sweep the brush in long, firm but gentle movements towards the heart. Once you have finished the left side of the body, continue in downward strokes along the right side, finishing at your right foot.

Remember to clean your body brush after each use. Washing in warm water with a few drops of tea tree oil will kill bacteria and rinse away the impurities that have been collected in the bristles.

exfoliating creams and gels

Like body brushing, beauty products that exfoliate the surface of the skin and remove accumulated dead skin cells can leave the skin feeling soft, smooth and completely pampered. Again, you should

regular exfoliation assists detoxification

always start at your left foot and work towards your heart in the same direction as your blood flow.

Be careful of products with harsh granules that can place stress on the skin and do more harm than good. The treatment should never hurt or irritate; it should gently pamper and relax while improving the texture of one of your most vital organs!

aromatherapy and essential oils

When combined with certain types of massage (in particular lymphatic-drainage techniques), the use of aromatherapy and essential oils may assist in stimulating the lymphatic system, thus aiding in the removal of toxins that contribute to the problem of cellulite.

The application of essential oils can also be very effective in hydrating and softening the skin and preventing early ageing, which may make the problem of cellulite seem less apparent.

certain essential oils can be beneficial to sluggish circulation

More importantly, the positive effect of essential oils on the psyche is invaluable, and twice daily applications of uplifting and stimulating blends can greatly improve your frame of mind, confidence and self-esteem. Try using a blend of four drops each of juniper berry and rosemary, and three drops each of cypress and patchouli in 30ml of a vegetable-derived carrier oil such as almond, wheatgerm or jojoba oil.

massage

Massage techniques that stimulate the circulatory and lymphatic systems such as lymphatic drainage can help to relieve the problem of cellulite. They have the ability to encourage sluggish circulation as well as assist in the elimination of toxins and wastes. A word of warning though: some techniques, such as deep tissue massage, can compound the problem. By massaging the problem spots of a person with poor lymph drainage and circulation in an intense way, the blood flow and lymph are stimulated. As the lymph drainage is poor to begin with, the toxins and wastes in the lymph simply collect between the fat cells of trouble zones.

Clearly, gentle massage techniques that gradually encourage circulation back to a healthy state are what is required, as they can help to reduce swelling and assist in smoothing the lumpiness of the tissues.

Massage will not, however, break down the fat cells in cellulite-affected areas. These can be tackled with a reduced fat intake and increased cardiovascular exercise once the problem of poor circulation has been addressed.

cellulite creams

There are many creams and lotions on the market tagged as cellulite cures. Formulas containing ingredients such as caffeine and other stimulants purport to be able to enter the bloodstream via the skin and assist in the fat elimination process. Others claim to have a remarkable toning and firming action on the skin, thereby reducing the appearance of cellulite on the hips, buttocks and thighs.

Most of these formulas contain incredibly nourishing moisturisers so, at the very least, they can relieve dry, scaly skin when used in conjunction with body brushing or exfoliation. For the most part, these creams and lotions contain quite luxurious formulations, so whether they act on your cellulite or not they will leave you feeling pampered and indulged. It's important to remember that the use of creams alone won't reduce your cellulite problem, however if you can afford it, they can be a lovely, luxurious part of your anti-cellulite program.

in-salon cellulite treatments

Let's be realistic here: A visit to the beauty salon leaves you feeling refreshed, relaxed and completely spoilt. While many women shun in-salon cellulite treatments, I find it hard to condemn them because at the very least the client receives a wonderfully pampering experience in a completely relaxing environment, and we all deserve to spoil ourselves regularly.

The key is not to go in expecting that an hour in a beauty salon will transform you into Elle MacPherson. Keep a realistic attitude about the results you will achieve and you won't be disappointed should you not drop a dress size after three visits.

In-salon treatments are usually designed by therapists who are very knowledgeable in their field, so if you choose to be indulged, expect careful and specific attention to problem areas, as well as head to toe pampering. Even if it has little effect on your cellulite, a visit to the salon will most likely leave you feeling pampered and gorgeous afterwards, and that can't be such a bad thing!

hydrotherapy and thallasotherapy

The use of water (hydrotherapy) and seaweed and marine extracts (thallasotherapy) in the elimination of toxins is nothing new, and is a common practice in many cultures. Advanced technology means that these practices are increasingly effective in helping to flush out wastes from the system and boost circulation. A hydrotherapy bath has several specifically aimed jets that massage the body in a defined routine from toe to head. Generally, the bath lasts about twenty to thirty minutes and nearly always leaves you feeling completely relaxed. How effective it is in reducing the appearance of cellulite is not clear, but it is known to provide a feeling of lightness, probably due to the flushing of the system.

Likewise, certain marine extracts and seaweed formulas have a high iodine content and so can have the ability to draw toxins from the body via the skin. When added to a bath they can assist in the removal of certain wastes. Again, whether these formulas have any radical effect on cellulite is unclear but, if nothing else, they do leave the skin feeling wonderfully clean and soft.

hydrotherapy baths stimulate lymphatic drainage and encourage detoxification

NOTE: It is recommended that pregnant women, people with high blood pressure, diabetes and/or a history of heart complaints avoid the use of essential oils unless under the supervision of a highly qualified and reputable aromatherapist. Likewise, pregnant women should steer clear of cellulite creams and in-salon treatments that raise the core body temperature such as wraps, hydrotherapy baths and detoxifying formulations. In cases of pregnancy and cosmetic use, most medical professionals recommend the old adage 'if in doubt, leave it out'. Indeed, a sure-fire recipe to a healthy, happy pregnancy is a simple, sensible and natural diet, lifestyle, and beauty regime.

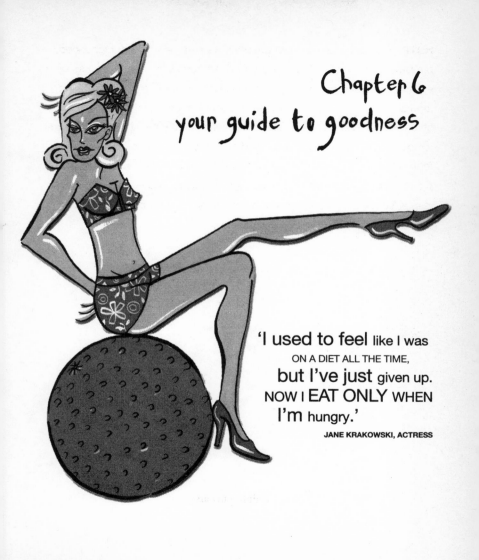

Chapter 6
your guide to goodness

'I used to feel like I was ON A DIET ALL THE TIME, but I've just given up. NOW I EAT ONLY WHEN I'm hungry.'

JANE KRAKOWSKI, ACTRESS

a simple, two-week detoxifying diet can be a great way to begin your anti-cellulite program. It will assist in stimulating the system, and allow the liver and kidneys to freely flush out impurities, without more toxins being added on a daily basis. Remember that this is not designed as a weight loss program. It is a cleansing, detoxifying program that will assist your body in eliminating wastes and impurities. Also keep in mind that after the two weeks, you can't simply go back to unhealthy eating habits and expect to maintain results. The idea is that this program will help you to develop sensible, healthy and good-for-you eating habits.

The following program, devised with the help of Anna Paredes from the Randwick Colon Care Centre in Sydney, is a gentle and effective two-week plan that will have you well on your way to a cleaner system. If at any time you feel hungry during this detoxification plan, reach for a healthy piece of fruit, such as a green apple or a pear, or some carrot or celery sticks. It may be hard for the first few days, but try to steer clear of tea, coffee, soft drinks and alcohol throughout the two-week program and, if possible, try to cut them out or at least reduce your intake once the two weeks is up. Try not to eat or drink after eight o'clock in the evening either, as this is your body's resting time. Wherever possible, opt for organic choices in all your foods. Finally, do not commence this or any other detoxifying program without first consulting your GP and a nutritionist.

week one

MORNING: Before showering, dry body brush for five minutes, starting at your left foot and working towards the heart. Follow with a warm shower and a cold rinse.

BREAKFAST: Squeeze the juice of half a lemon into a glass of pure, hot water and drink. Follow immediately with two large glasses of pure, room temperature water. Cut up half a papaya, a medium-sized kiwi fruit and a few slices of pineapple or a pear into a salad and top with three tablespoons of sheep or goat's milk yoghurt and a sprinkle of LSA (linseed, sunflower seeds and almond meal ground up). If you are vegan use soy-derived yoghurt.

DETOXIFYING JUICE: Three carrots, half a beetroot, two leaves of spinach, one green apple and a small knob of ginger.

MORNING TEA: One cup of dandelion or green tea and one green apple or a pear.

LUNCH: Three glasses of pure, room temperature water with a little squeeze of lemon in each glass. A medium-sized piece of grilled fish or skinless chicken with a large rocket salad, sunflower seeds, olive oil and lemon juice. One large vegetable juice, e.g. carrot, celery, ginger, and beetroot.

SNACK: Ten raw almonds and one green apple or a pear followed by a cup of green or dandelion tea.

DINNER: Three glasses of pure, room temperature water with a little squeeze of lemon in each glass. Half a cup of brown rice with a medium-sized piece of fish or skinless chicken (grilled) or two small lamb chops (grilled). Slice two cucumbers diagonally with your meal. If vegan or vegetarian, replace the meat or fish with tofu, zucchini, eggplant and mushrooms.

Or Vegetable soup with beans and brown rice.

Or One egg omelette with mushrooms or zucchini.

AFTER DINNER: Cut four small pieces of ginger, place into a pot or glass of hot water and leave for twenty minutes then drink while still hot to speed metabolism and aid digestion.

BEFORE BED DETOXIFYING BATH: Mix one quarter of a cup of Epsom salts and almond oil into a scrub. Massage over entire body, in circular motions, focusing on the abdominal region, the thighs and the buttocks. Avoid the face. Submerge yourself into a hot bath with 250g of Epsom salts for a maximum of twenty minutes. Any longer can mean that your body reabsorbs the toxins the bath has stimulated to release.

week two

MORNING: Dry body brushing as in week one.

BREAKFAST: Drink one glass of pure, hot water and lemon juice followed by two glasses of pure, room temperature water. Cut up half a papaya, a medium-sized kiwi fruit and a few slices of pineapple or a pear into a salad and top with three tablespoons of sheep or goat's milk yoghurt and a sprinkle of LSA (linseed, sunflower seeds and almond meal ground up). If you are vegan use soy-derived yoghurt.

MORNING TEA: One cup of dandelion or green tea. One green apple or an orange.

LUNCH: One large vegetable juice combination (as in week one). Large rocket salad with grilled fish or skinless chicken, and one quarter of an avocado with olive oil and lemon juice.

SNACK: One banana, ten raw almonds, and one cup of green or dandelion tea.

DINNER: Three glasses of pure, room temperature water with a little squeeze of lemon in each glass. Soup made from carrots, celery, tomatoes, shaved beetroot, lentils and brown rice with a small amount of sea salt or Celtic salt (they contain many minerals our bodies need).

Or   Brown rice with either grilled chicken, fish, lamb chops or tofu, with goat's cheese, vegetables, and tahini as your dressing.

Or   Small pumpkin soup with parsley followed by one baked sweet potato.

AFTER DINNER: Ginger tea or Chi tea.

BEFORE BED DETOXIFYING BATH: Continue with the detoxifying scrub and bath as in week one, for up to six to eight weeks.

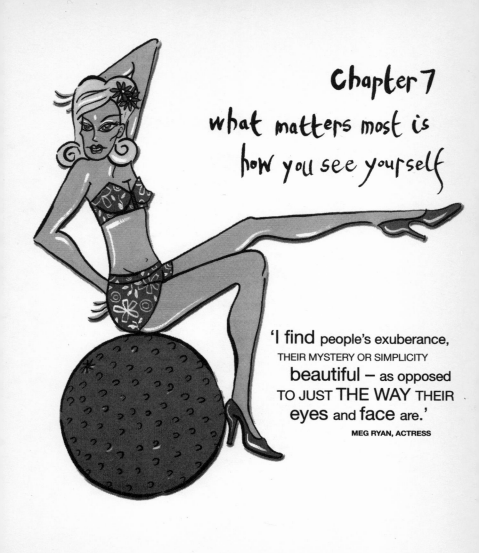

Chapter 7

what matters most is how you see yourself

'I find people's exuberance, THEIR MYSTERY OR SIMPLICITY beautiful – as opposed TO JUST THE WAY THEIR eyes and face are.'

MEG RYAN, ACTRESS

much of the way other people perceive us comes from our own perception of self – from our self-esteem and the way we feel deep inside. This is usually reflected in the way we stand, walk, talk, sit, and generally hold ourselves. It's true that something like cellulite can be depressing and can lower your self-esteem dramatically, but it really doesn't need to. There is no reason on earth why any woman should feel less feminine, less beautiful or less worthy of praise and attention simply because she has a few lumps and bumps.

I know of extremely successful models who grace the covers of magazines and are hailed as

exercise helps boost self-esteem

the most beautiful women in the world who suffer from cellulite. It may get them down, but you would never guess. Okay, they may have the advantage of personal stylists, clever lighting and computers that can 'fix' problem areas so their legs and bottoms always look smooth and sexy on magazine covers, but that doesn't solve the problem in real life.

The secret these women have is that they have learnt how to play up their best features, and how to disguise their faults, or even make whatever figure or facial 'fault' they have work to their advantage. In doing so, these women have developed that inner self-confidence and poise that is the key to true beauty.

Try to take a balanced approach to beauty. I know this is often hard, especially when your attention is centred on a particular trouble spot. Look at your body as a whole, not just the sum of its parts. Don't focus on a double chin, dimply thighs or child bearing hips, focus on how fabulous and strong your shoulders are, or how healthy and shiny your hair is, or how sparkling and lively your eyes are. Instead of spending all your efforts trying to cover up the bits you don't like, enhance and highlight the features you do like. Celebrate your shoulders and a fabulous bust in elegant necklines that subtly draw attention to this area. Wear your hair in a way that will show off its lustre, or learn tricks with make-up colours to bring out the colour and definition of your eyes.

Exercise is a fabulous self-esteem booster. Aside from the rush you get each time you work out, after a month or so of thrice weekly workouts, you will notice the beginnings of muscle definition. Your posture will improve and your skin tone will radiate. Soon you will exercise not just to lose weight or tone up, but simply because it makes you feel amazing.

There is also nothing like a great outfit to boost your confidence. A little bit of savvy shopping and sensible daily wardrobe choices can really help. When you know you have your presentation spot-on, you inevitably feel great and can easily project a more confident self to the world.

a well-made classy heel can create a sleek, elegant leg

If cellulite is a concern for you, try a few fashion tricks to disguise the problem until your cellulite-reducing program starts to work. Darker colours worn on the lower half of the body tend to slim this area down and create a leaner silhouette. Quality fabrics cut with longer lines and simple designs do the same. There's also nothing like a really classy pair of beautifully shaped heels to create a sleek, elegant leg. Add a pair of silky pantihose in the same colour to enhance the look.

There are some golden rules you should adhere to if you want to disguise cellulite or heavier legs. These include:

- Always wear the same colour pantihose as your shoes and, in this case, make sure both the hosiery and your shoes match the colour of your skirt or pants exactly.
- Aim to avoid tight-fitting clothes, cheaper fabrics that may not sit well on the body, and fussy, frilly finishes.
- Try to wear longer lines in skirts and dresses that have a classic, elegant shape. Short skirts can emphasise the problem, as can fuller skirts. For the same reason, avoid wearing pants with full pockets, pleating, or that are clingy and tight.

Fashion and beauty tips aside, the best thing you can do for your self-esteem is to be the best person you can. Respect yourself. Try to think pure, healthy thoughts. Find the time to be kind to others – it's a great way to feel good about yourself. Even if it's something as small as paying someone a compliment, when you do something that improves another person's day, or their frame of mind, that good feeling can't help but rub off on you.

Conversely, the more you bring other people down or criticise them, the more you are beating yourself up. Bringing another person down is not the way to raise your own self-esteem and confidence; rather, it actually has the effect of lowering your self-esteem. Negativity breeds negativity and you end up feeling unhappy and ugly on the inside.

Most importantly remember that true beauty is inner beauty. It shines through in an act of kindness, a smile and a laugh, self-confidence and compassion. Take time out to get to know yourself. Be good to yourself on every level – physically, mentally, emotionally and spiritually. Pretty soon your cellulite won't seem like such an insurmountable problem.

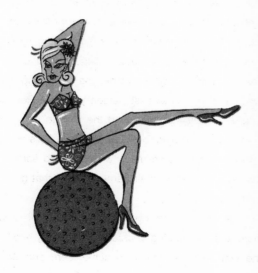

what matters most is how you see yourself   73

bibliography

Chopra, D. *Creating Health – How to Wake Up the Body's Intelligence*, rev. edn, HarperCollins, London, 1996.

Eats, T. & Cook, G. *The Complete Guide to Health and Well-Being*, Lansdowne, Sydney, 1998.

Lamm, S. *Younger at Last*, Simon & Schuster, New York, 1998.

Lanctot, G. *Great Legs, How to Have Them at Any Age*, Sidgwick & Jackson, London, 1988.

Martin-Wurwand, J. *Cellulite, A Reality Check*, Dermascope Newsletter, The International Dermal Institute, USA, 1996.

Michalun, N. & Michalun, M.V. *Milady's Skin Care and Cosmetics Dictionary*, Milady Publishing Company, New York, 1994.

Sturt, C. *Beauty, Skin and Self-Esteem*, Nacson & Sons, Sydney, 1998.

Tierra, M. *The Way of Chinese Herbs*, Simon & Schuster, Australia, 1998.

Winter, R. *A Consumer's Dictionary of Cosmetic Ingredients*, Crown, New York, 1989.

Also available from Vermilion:

The Raw Energy Bible

Leslie Kenton

When Leslie and Susannah Kenton's Raw Energy was first published, it became an instant bestseller. A Raw Energy way of eating – in which 50 to 75 per cent of your foods are taken raw – can bring natural weight loss without dieting, help prevent colds and flu, rejuvenate the body in medically measurable ways, enhance athletic performance, heighten energy and bring greater mental clarity and emotional balance.

Recent biochemical research into the powerful antioxidant, health protective effects of raw fruits and vegetables has added another piece to the mysterious puzzle of how Raw Energy works its wonders.

A unique compilation of the bestselling titles *Raw Energy Food Combining Diet, Raw Energy Recipes* and *Juice High, The Raw Energy Bible* combines this new material with practical information, techniques and recipes, producing the ultimate Raw Energy sourcebook to help you revolutionise your own health and good looks.

Buy Vermilion Books

Order further Vermilion titles from your local bookshop, or have them delivered direct to your door by Bookpost

☐ **The Raw Energy Bible** by Leslie Kenton   0091856647   £6.99
☐ **Detox Now** by Leslie Kenton   0091825822   £3.99
☐ **The Luscious Low-fat Cookbook**
    by Alison Rose & Tony Guy   0091882834   £10.99
☐ **The Core Programme** by Peggy Brill   0091882419   £9.99
☐ **New Vital Oils** by Liz Earle   0091876699   £7.99
☐ **Beauty Fixes** by Josephine Fairley   0091882230   £7.99
☐ **Feel Good Naked** by Laure Redmond   0091884187   £6.99

FREE POST AND PACKING
Overseas customers allow £2 per paperback

PHONE: 01624 677237

POST: Random House Books
c/o Bookpost, PO Box 29, Douglas
Isle of Man, IM99 1BQ

FAX: 01624 670923

EMAIL: bookshop@enterprise.net

Cheques and credit cards accepted

Prices and availability subject to change without notice.
Allow 28 days for delivery.

www.randomhouse.co.uk